YOUR KNOWLEDGE HAS VALUE

Bibliographic information published by the German National Library:

The German National Library lists this publication in the National Bibliography; detailed bibliographic data are available on the Internet at http://dnb.dnb.de .

Imprint:

Copyright © 2020 GRIN Verlag
Print and binding: Books on Demand GmbH, Norderstedt Germany
ISBN: 9783346219428

This book at GRIN:

https://www.grin.com/document/900993

Sara Vincenzotti

Admission of a mental disabled people to institutional care. Effective protection or arbitrary detention?

GRIN Verlag

GRIN - Your knowledge has value

Since its foundation in 1998, GRIN has specialized in publishing academic texts by students, college teachers and other academics as e-book and printed book. The website www.grin.com is an ideal platform for presenting term papers, final papers, scientific essays, dissertations and specialist books.

Visit us on the internet:

http://www.grin.com/

http://www.facebook.com/grincom

http://www.twitter.com/grin_com

1) Critically evaluate the extent to which the law relating to the admission of people with a mental disability to institutional care provides effective protection of the right to protection from arbitrary detention.

Introduction

The aim of this essay is to critically evaluate the development of procedural safeguards regarding deprivation of incapacitated patients' liberty in institutional care. It will assess the extent to which the law is successful in protecting patients' rights against arbitrary detention, and led to the conclusion that neither the past law nor the current law have adequately safeguarded people's rights against arbitrary detainment. To do so, it will start by evaluating the development of the protection of liberty frameworks in the UK, and how their inadequacy led to the implementation of DOLS in hospitals and care homes. Consequently, there will be an evaluation of three main criticisms. Firstly, it will look at the level of complexity of DOLS, both on a politico-legal plane and on a practical medical plane. Secondly, it will look at what is held to constitute as a deprivation of liberty, and how there are significant gaps in this definition. Thirdly, it will take a closer look at the implications of the *Cheshire West*[1] judgment and evaluate the consequences of broadening the scope for DOLS. This essay will thus reach the conclusion that the law relating to the admission of incapacitated patients has failed to properly assess individuals' rights to protection from arbitrary detention.

Development of the Protection of Liberty Framework

The Mental Capacity Act 2005 (MCA) as well as the Mental Health Act 1983 (MHA) contain various statutory provisions aimed at protecting the liberty of individuals suffering from mental disabilities. The MHA established such a framework to provide medical treatment on both a voluntary and involuntary basis, these would either be achieved by formal or informal detention measures.[2] The MCA on the other hand, provides a framework specifically for incapacitated patients.[3] Prior to the passing of the MCA, this

---

[1] *Cheshire West and Chester Council v P [2014]* UKSC 19.
[2] MHA 1983, Sections 131, and 2-3.
[3] Richardson, 'Mental capacity at the margin: the interface between two Acts' (2010) 18 Medical Law Review 1, 57.

area caused various predicaments for the courts. This was due to informal admissions under such circumstances leaving patients without any of the formal safeguards which are in place to protect patients in compulsory detention.[4] The lack of formal safeguards meant that many incapacitated patients were being detained in hospitals and care homes with no rights to protect them from arbitrary detention.

Before the MCA was implemented, patients who lacked capacity were often accommodated in hospitals under common law resources, so as not to require formal detention schemes via the MHA.[5] This was proven to be arbitrary and in breach of a patients' human rights in the landmark case of *HL*,[6] which will be further discussed throughout this essay. As the MHA and common law doctrine was unable to adequately protect incapacitated patients' rights, Parliament development a framework under the MCA 2005 known as deprivation of liberty safeguards (DOLS). This framework intended to give incapacitated individuals a certain degree of protection safeguards. The DOLS provided a framework which lawfully justified the deprivation of a person's liberty in a hospital or care home, under specific circumstances which had been authorised by a supervisory body.[7] Despite this attempt, DOLS have been described as 'an administrative and bureaucratic nightmare',[8] with the Select Committee rendering them 'not fit for purpose' less than five years after being implemented.[9]

Prior to the MCA 2005, compliant yet incapacitated patients would often be informally detained in hospital under the common law, namely the doctrines of necessity and best interests established in *West Berkshire*.[10] The use of the common law in such a way came under question in the case of *Bournewood*,[11] where an autistic and profoundly mentally

---

[4] Jackson, E., *Medical Law: Texts, Cases and Materials* (5th ed) (OUP, 2019), 364.

[5] Richardson, *opt cit* note 3, 58.

[6] *HL v The United Kingdom [2004] (2005) 40 EHRR 32.*

[7] Dwyer, S., 'The Deprivation of Liberty Safeguards and People with Dementia: Implications for Social Workers' (2010) British Journal of Social Work 40, 1503-1516, 1503.

[8] Keene, A.R., 'Mental Capacity Report: Special Report: the Law Commission's Mental Capacity and Deprivation of Liberty Report (Law Com No. 372)' (2017) *39 Essex Chambers*, 2.

[9] House of Lords Paper 139, *Select Committee on the Mental Capacity Act 2005*, 'Mental Capacity Act 2005: post-legislative scrutiny' Report of Session 2013–14, para 32.

[10] *F v West Berkshire Health Authority and another [1989] 2 All ER 545.*

[11] *R. v Bournewood Community and Mental Health NHS Trust Ex p. L [1998] UKHL 24.*

incapacitated man had been detained in hospital after becoming agitated at a day centre. The hospital denied his carers to visit the ward under fear that he would want to leave, which led his carers to bring the case to court for wrongful confinement. When the case reached the House of Lords, they referred back to *West Berkshire*, and held that any confinement would be justified by the inherent jurisdiction of the Court.[12] The House of Lords judgment resulted in the 'Bournewood gap', which became known as 'the lack of legal procedure for a person who lacked capacity to seek a review of their detention for care or treatment'.[13] The *Bournewood* gap resulted in much criticism, with the Law Commission stating the law was 'unsystematic and full of glaring gaps',[14] as well as Lord Steyn held this statutory failure as an 'indefensible gap in [UK] mental health law'.[15]

These criticisms emphasised the significant lack of procedural safeguards for incapacitated mentally disabled patients. However, it was not until the case was brought to the European Court of Human Rights (ECtHR) in 2004 that real change occurred. The appeal was launched to assess whether there had been a violation of the right to liberty under Article 5 of the European Convention of Human Rights (ECHR), which states that 'no one shall be deprived of his liberty save in ... accordance with a procedure prescribed by law',[16] with subsection 1(e) specifying instances of the lawful detention of people of 'unsound mind'.[17] Article 5 placed heavy emphasis on procedures that must be in place to establish adequate safeguards in order to protect arbitrary detention, as well as the right to challenge a deprivation of liberty in Court. The ECtHR held that the UK was in breach of Article 5(1) and 5(4), as there were no procedures in place which assessed the legality of detentions, nor were individuals given the opportunity to dispute the detention in Court.[18] The first case heard in the ECtHR regarding persons of unsound mind was

---

[12] Bartlett, P., and Sandland, R., *Mental Health Law: Policy and Practice* (4th ed) (OUP, 2013), 204.
[13] Pearce, N., and Jackson., S., 'Deprivation of Liberty Safeguards Part 2: the Authorisation Regime: statutory provisions of authorisations and Code of Practice' (April, 2012) Fam Law 432, 432.
[14] Law Commission Report, Mental Incapacity (Law Com No. 231) [1995], Para 1.1
[15] *R. v Bournewood Community and Mental Health NHS Trust Ex p. L [1997] EWCA 2879.*
[16] Article 5(1) ECHR.
[17] Article 5(1)(e) ECHR.
[18] *HL v The United Kingdom [2004] (2005) 40 EHRR 32.*

that of *Winterwrep*[19] in 1979, which established certain requirements for detention. The Strasbourg court held that the 'unsoundness of mind' must follow from a 'true mental disorder' which has been determined by an 'objective medical expert',[20] and that the disorder must be 'of a kind or degree warranting compulsory confinement'.[21] The *Winterwerp* requirements go hand in hand with the ECHR Article 5 requirements, and must be taken to mean that a judgement must be 'consistent with the express and implied principles of the ECHR as a whole, being fair and proper, and protecting the individual from arbitrariness'.[22] The court went even further in an attempt to define a deprivation of liberty, and used the 1981 Italian Mafia case of *Guzzardi*[23] to reiterate that a deprivation did not simply constitute a prohibition of physical movement, but demanded an assessment of 'the type, duration, effects and manner of implementation of the measures in question'.[24]

Having applied these already existing legal principles, the ECtHR held that even if there was no breach of English domestic law in *HL*, the UK was in breach of Article 5 by not providing effective safeguards. In fact, Article 5 rights specifically disregarded whether the patient manifested a desire to leave the institution,[25] and consequently the House of Lords could not use HL's compliance to mean his detention was lawful. The substantial extent of control executed by clinicians over HL's movements, care and contact with family marked a particular 'degree and intensity of control',[26] which led to the conclusion that he had been unlawfully detained. Further, the court held that there was a 'striking .. lack of any fixed procedural rules by which the admission and detention of compliant incapacitated persons [was] conducted', and that it noted a particular 'lack of any formalised admission procedures which indicate who can propose admission, for what

---

[19] *Winterwerp v the Netherlands* (Application No. 6301/73) [1979] 2 EHRR 387.
[20] *Ibid*, para 39.
[21] *Ibid*.
[22] Bartlett, *opt cit* note 12, 206.
[23] *Guzzardi v Italy (Application no. 7367/76)* [1981] 3 E.H.R.R. 333.
[24] *Ibid*, para 92.
[25] *HL v The United Kingdom [2004] (2005) 40 EHRR 32*, para 90.
[26] Keywood, K., 'Detaining Mentally Disordered Patients Lacking Capacity: The arbitrariness of informal detention and the common law doctrine of necessity' (2005) Med Law Rev, 110.

reasons and on the basis of what kind of medical .. assessments'.[27] The court thus concluded that the limited level of jurisprudence regarding the meaning and application of the best interest test[28] proves that there were no substantive rules, and held that the doctrine used by the UK courts was devoid of the necessary procedural safeguards required to ensure the *Winterwerp* criteria was being correctly enforced.[29] This meant that there was no legal measures relating to the protection of the right to liberty against arbitrary admission of incapacitated patients. The violation of Article 5 led the UK government to introduce a safeguard framework specifically for regulating deprivations of liberty of incapacitated individuals. This led to the amendment of the MCA 2005 to include the deprivation of liberty safeguards (DOLS), which will now be evaluated.

MCA 2005 and the Deprivation of Liberty Safeguards

The amendments brought by the Mental Health Act 2007 introduced Schedule A1 and 1A to the MCA 2005. The process by which DOLS is applied neatly follows the *Winterwerp* criteria. Schedule A1 introduced six categories, which must all be satisfied in order to obtain an authorisation to deprive a person of their liberty:

1) The person must be at least 18 years of age;

2) The person must suffer from a mental disorder as defined by the MHA 1983[30] and there must have been a medical assessment of the person by an approved doctor;[31]

3) The person must lack capacity to decide whether they wish to be admitted in institutional care;[32]

4) The institution must establish that the person's detention is in their best interest, and that the degree of detention is proportionate to the likelihood and severity of harm;[33]

---

[27] *HL v The United Kingdom [2004] (2005) 40 EHRR 32,* para 120.
[28] Bartlett, *opt cit* note 12, 207.
[29] Keywood, *opt cit* note 26, 111.
[30] MCA 2005, Schedule A1, Part 3, para 14.
[31] Mental Capacity Act 2005: Code of Practice (2007) (TSO, London), para 4.35-39.
[32] Sections 1-3, MCA 2005.
[33] MCA 2005, Schedule A1, Part 3, para 16.

5) The person must satisfy the relevant eligibility, therefore meaning they cannot be assessed under DOLS if they are already subject to MHA 1983 provisions;[34]

6) An assessment into whether the person has made an effective and valid advance decision refusing the treatment in question, which would make detainment for treatment and care unlawful.[35]

Further procedural safeguards are found in the necessity of periodic reviews of the type of detention, as well as the appointing of a representative to survey all procedures and the patient's overall management.[36] In addition, the MCA established the Court of Protection, which allowed for incapacitated patients or their representative to challenge their detention.[37] These safeguards require formal assessments to be made by the relevant supervisory bodies, therefore once they are satisfied with the requirements, the deprivation of a patient's liberty is justified under law *if* it is in their best interest to be detained.[38] Schedule A1 also sets out the relevant procedures for the institution's managing authority to obtain the required authorisation to deprive a patient of their liberty. As per the DOL Code of Practice, managing authorities have a duty to identify whether depriving a patient of his liberty is necessary, whether all practical steps have been taken to determine if the deprivation is necessary, and whether all reasonable and practical steps have been taken to avoid depriving them of their liberty.[39] If the managing authority believes a patient is being deprived, or will be deprived of his liberty, they have the duty to request a supervisory body for an authorisation to do so.[40] The supervisory body must then appoint assessors to each of the six qualifying requirements, and pay particular attention to appointing different assessors for the best interest and mental health valuation.[41] The supervisory body must also ensure that either a family member or an Independent Mental Capacity Advocate is appointed to consult regarding the patient's

---

[34] MCA 2005, Schedule A1, Part 3, para 17.
[35] Pearce, N., and Jackson., S., *opt cit* note 13.
[36] Section 39, MCA 2005.
[37] Section 45, MCA 2005.
[38] Banner, N., 'The Bournewood Gap and the Deprivation of Liberty Safeguards in the Mental Capacity Act 2005' (2011) 18 Philosophy, Psychiatry, & Psychology 2, 123-126.
[39] Code of Practice (2007), *opt cit* note 31, para 3.6.
[40] Pearce, N., and Jackson., S., *opt cit* note 13, 432.
[41] *Ibid*, 436.

best interests, as well as to be appointed to assist the patient during his commitment.[42] It therefore seems clear that the introduction of DOLS results in a number of hurdles which need to be passed, and Parliament's intention in including them was to add safeguards. However, they have not been successful in doing so. The DOLS framework is 'overly complex', 'not well understood' and 'poorly implemented',[43] which makes the scheme nothing more than a bureaucratic nightmare.[44] To assess the reasons behind the failure of the DOLS framework, I will now evaluate why they have been deemed unsuccessful.

Unnecessary Complexity and Draconian Language

When describing what judging a DOLS case was like, Charles J held it was 'as if you [had] been in a washing machine and spin dryer'.[45] Similarly, Lady Hale said that 'the safeguards have the appearance of bewildering complexity',[46] making them widely impenetrable by lay people. This is a significant problem for the implementation of DOLS, as it means institutions often need expert legal advice to understand their duties and the necessary procedures. This is particularly worrying for small care homes, which are left 'marooned with all the responsibility' to apply for the specified authorisation with a severe lack of guidance.[47] The complexity of Schedule A1 imposes 'an enormous administrative burden' on understaffed and undertrained local authorities, as well as draining an already over stretched budget.[48] As the process is so inherently complex, it is not surprising that local authorities have raised difficulties in their implementation. This is in direct correlation with the reality that local authorities and small care homes often attempt to make shortcuts or ways to avoid going through the procedures,[49] which proves that DOLS do not effectively protect the right to liberty, but rather simply serve as a bureaucratic measure.

---

[42] Bartlett, P., *opt cit* note 12, 209.
[43] HoL 139, *opt cit* note 9, page 7.
[44] Keene, R:, *opt cit* note 8, 2.
[45] Jackson, *opt cit* note 4, 370.
[46] *Cheshire West and Chester Council v P [2014] UKSC 19, [2014] MHLO 16.*
[47] Pearce, N., and Jackson., S., 'Deprivation of Liberty Safeguards Part 6: definition of deprivation of liberty' (August, 2012) Fam Law 999, 999.
[48] Pearce, N., and Jackson., S., 'Deprivation of Liberty Safeguards Part 3: how the authorisation regime safeguards are working' (May, 2012) Fam Law 567, 567.
[49] *Ibid.*

The overlay of different regulations and guidelines leads to further problems of application. The DOLS Code of Practice notes that those covered under the scheme suffer from 'significant learning disabilities', neurological conditions such as brain damage, or older patients often suffering from dementia.'[50] The reality however, is that these conditions all require very different care and treatment, therefore, putting them all under the umbrella of a single scheme is not very effective. For example, individuals with learning disabilities have been described as having a 'complex history culminating in a crisis'.[51] Patients with autism, or Down Syndrome have always had a specific way of life, mostly fixed in routine and coping mechanisms. This is widely different from an 80 year old patient admitted with dementia. Stewart notes how relatively unprotected people with dementia can be, stating that many 'are admitted permanently against their will to institutional facilities because of pressure from families and on the say-so of a single doctor'.[52] In order to adequately protect the rights of each patient, social workers must have a particularly high level of awareness about not only everyday practice, but also their legal responsibilities.[53]

As Blamires noted in her study of care homes, an interviewee held they would always consult with other professionals, including those working in their local DOLS offices, as many staff members did not have the confidence to 'go straight in' and make an application.[54] Similarly, another interviewee noted that the 'systems are great in principle, but you need people there to implement them' which they held to be widely unavailable in out-of-area placements and learning disability hospitals.[55] This is further proof that the environment in which care homes, hospitals and local authorities operate in terms of DOLS, is 'not legally coherent and bristles with intricate regulations' that staff does not feel comfortable applying.[56] The lack of understanding of guidelines and procedures by

---

[50] Code of Practice (2007), *opt cit* note 31, para 1.7.
[51] Blamires, K., Forrester-Jones, R., and Murphy, G., 'An Investigation into the use of the Deprivation of Liberty Safeguards with People with Intellectual Disabilities' (2017) Journal of Applied Research in Intellectual Disabilities 30, 714-726, 720.
[52] Stewart, R., 'Letter' (2006) *British Medical Journal 332*, 118–19.
[53] Dwyer, S., '*opt cit* note 7, 1506.
[54] Blamires, K., *opt cit* note 51, 720.
[55] *Ibid*, 719.
[56] Pearce, N., and Jackson., S., *opt cit* note 48, 567.

medical staff, along with the inherent complexity of the procedure itself, fails to keep incapacitated adults safe. The priority, which should be safeguarding a patient's right to liberty, becomes clouded by the highly bureaucratic and administrative procedures needed to authorise DOLS.

No Definition of Deprivation of Liberty

The trigger for the DOLS process is the belief that a patient is being, or will need to be, deprived of their liberty. The MCA[57] defines a deprivation of liberty simply by quoting the meaning from the ECHR's Article 5.[58] The problem of doing this, is that Article 5 does not actually define what a deprivation of liberty constitutes. It simply notes how and when one should not deprive an individual of their liberty. This creates a large gap in the law, which makes it infinitely hard to use as a shield against the deprivation of liberty when we do not actually know what we should regard as one. In order to rectify this, the UK took to common law to define a deprivation of liberty. *Bournewood* already told us that the central question around a deprivation of liberty was whether the patient lacking capacity was free to leave institutional care.[59] Further, it was specified as an objective hypothetical test. Whether the patient had tried to leave or expressed they wanted to leave, was irrelevant to the test of deprivation. The focus was only on the *reaction* the care institution would have if they did.[60] This was further emphasised in the Supreme Court's decision on *Cheshire West,* where Lady Hale noted that 'a gilded cage is still a cage'.[61] This thus developed what is now known as the acid test, which assessed whether the patient was under continuous and complete supervision or control, and whether they were free to leave care of their own free will.[62] The acid test joined in the Court of Appeal's firstly developed three stage test. Firstly, there needs to be an objective element of the individual's confinement, to a specific institution for a non-negotiable amount of time.[63] An account must be taken of a varied list of criteria, such as 'type, duration, effects and

[57] Section 64(5), MCA 2005
[58] Article 5(1), ECHR
[59] Jackson, E., *opt cit* note 4, 365.
[60] *Ibid.*
[61] *Cheshire West and Chester Council v P [2014] UKSC 19,* para 46.
[62] Clements, 'Disability, Dignity and the cri de coeur' (2011) EHRLR 675.
[63] Bartlett, P., *opt cit* note 12, 214.

manner of implementation'.[64] Secondly, a subjective element, which lies in the individual's inability to give valid consent to the confinement. And thirdly, the deprivation in question must be one originating from the State.[65] The pressure put on the State by this requirement intended to broaden their responsibility beyond not breaching Article 5, but to include a 'positive obligation' to protect liberty.[66] However, due to the procedural aspects of the DOLS, this pressure is felt by local authorities and managing authorities of institutional care. The issue with this is that these parties are not equipped to deal with common law jurisdictions, and therefore leaves them with a highly disorganised framework and vague guideline to deprivation of liberty assessments. It is therefore not a stretch to say that the lack of a clear definition fails to provide appropriate safeguards to patients, as often clinicians and care workers simply do not know what they are looking for.[67] This has been noted by research conducted by Selmes et al, who found that clinicians were often very anxious about having to apply legal principles addressed in case law into the real life clinical cases.[68] The study also showed clinicians had a clear difficulty defining and understanding what constitutes a deprivation of liberty,[69] which again proves that they are simply not equipped to deal with such a chaotic law heavy framework.

In addition, the use of the common law as a means to develop a definition of deprivations of liberties is largely ineffective when necessary to educate a selection of lay people on the meaning. Richardson points out that decision makers like managing authorities and their staff are being confronted with multiple factors deciphered in case law which must be considered, yet they are given no guidance of priority levels nor how to achieve such assessments.[70] The Code of Practice only adds to the confusion, stating that the use of physical or chemical restraints could be signs of deprivations of liberty and that all less

---

[64] Allen, N., 'Restricting Movement or Depriving Liberty?' (2009) *Journal of Mental Health Law*, 23.
[65] *Cheshire West and Chester Council v P [2011]* EWCA Civ 1257, para 16.
[66] *Stanev v Bulgaria (Application No. 36760/06)* [2012] ECHR 46, para 118.
[67] Richardson, *opt cit* note 3, 76.
[68] Selmes, T., *et al*, "Prevalence of deprivation of liberty: a survey of in-patient services" (2010) *34 The Psychiatrist 6*, 221-5.
[69] *Ibid.*
[70] Richardson, *opt cit* note 3, 75.

restrictive methods must be used prior to admission.[71] However, in Munby LJ's judgement of *Cheshire West*, he held that 'restraint by itself is not deprivation of liberty'.[72] Similarly, the use of the least restrictive method places care homes under quite a large question mark. The *Cheshire West* judgment as well as the Code of Practice places an important emphasis on the patient's own context and specific circumstances, however, they also give undue reliance on the alternative methods available to institutions. Often local authorities are already underfunded and over stretched, therefore options are a luxury. If a patient objects to living in a particular ward or finds supervision intrusive, managing authorities will often not count it as a deprivation as there is no realistic alternative to give the patient.[73] This is incredibly important. Since it is the managing authority's responsibility to refer cases to a supervisory body to review placement, if they do not believe there are any deprivations then there simply will be no recourse to the DOLS,[74] and instead will be up to the patient's representative to challenge the detention in the Court of Protection. The lack of a statutory definition of what constitutes as a deprivation of liberty, in conjunction with repetitive, over-complicated and contradictory guidance, is a clear sign of DOLS' failure to adequately safeguard patients' rights to liberty. By not equipping medical staff and local authorities with guidelines and procedures built on clarity and conciseness, Parliament is severely impacting their ability to protect patients from arbitrary detention.

The Broadening of Deprivations of Liberty and its Consequences

The *Cheshire West* judgement significantly impacted the number of people potentially affected by DOLS. The broadening of the scope of deprivations of liberty was essentially a policy decision, taken by the Supreme Court to ensure there is always independent scrutiny to protect vulnerable people in care. This can be seen in Lady Hale's judgment, where she noted the imperative need for 'periodic independent checks' on a patients' arrangements in relation to their best interests.[75] This new surge of power to the patients

---

[71] Code of Practice (2008) *opt cit* note 31, para 2.5 and 2.7.
[72] *Cheshire West and Chester Council v P [2011]* EWCA Civ 1257, para 23.
[73] Pearce, N., and Jackson., S., *opt cit* note 471004.
[74] *Ibid.*
[75] *Cheshire West and Chester Council v P [2014]* UKSC 19, para 57.

and their representatives led to an often automatic application for DOLS, due to the realisation that virtually any action taken by a care institution could be construed as amounting to a deprivation of liberty.[76] As *Guzzardi* has taught us, deprivation of liberty goes far beyond the restriction of movement, and should instead be an assessment of the degree and intensity of one's restrictions, rather than the nature of substance.[77] This also significantly broadened the scope of assessment. Allen argued that determining whether a deprivation of liberty has occurred under such a wide-ranging standard is not an 'easy task', due to the many borderline cases which are often a matter of opinion.[78]

A further set of consequences of the expansion, are the practical and financial implication of *Cheshire West*. Numerous NHS bodies commented on the increased backlog of cases; elevated numbers of authorisation referrals not being assessed, due to the high pressure of cases and low staffing issues; the impractical legal time scales, which do not coincide with the medical sphere and thus are often breached; and perhaps most prominently, staff shortage for qualified and experienced roles, who not only understand the surface of DOLS, but know how to implement them accurately.[79] It therefore seems clear that the current framework is too broadly implemented, especially given that the standard that is being implemented (deprivation of liberty) is not actually defined in any clear way. This makes DOLS not suitable for practice, and although its procedures have the clear intention of protecting patients from arbitrary detention, it fails to do so.

Concluding Remarks

After an evaluation of DOLS, it seems clear that the current framework is 'in crisis and needs to be overhauled'.[80] The current system is hectic, unorganised and unnecessarily complex. Going through the DOLS process has been identified by families as deeply distressing, and providing practically no protection for incapacitated adults.[81] The

---

[76] Pearce, N., and Jackson., S., 'Deprivation of Liberty Safeguards Part 5: general jurisdiction and role of the Court of Protection' (July, 2012) Fam Law 851, 851.
[77] *Guzzardi v Italy (Application no. 7367/76)* [1981] 3 E.H.R.R. 333.
[78] Allen, N., *opt cit* note 64, 22.
[79] Keene, A.R., *opt cit* note 8 2.
[80] *Ibid.*
[81] *Ibid.*, 3.

procedural aspects of the framework are 'voluminous, badly drafted, overly bureaucratic, and hard to understand'.[82] The reality is that if clinicians do not know how to implement DOLS, they cannot protect individuals from arbitrary detention. The dramatic increase in applications and court hearings instigated by DOLS is not evidence of progress, it is evidence of an ineffective system. Equally, the use of draconian language throughout Schedule A1 does not fit the rest of the MCA, which is successful in putting patients' autonomy first, and taking a modern approach to medical treatment. The judgment in *Cheshire West*, despite its good intentions, has only made patients' rights to liberty harder to identify and protect, due to the unnecessary broad scope filtered in. Therefore, there is no difficulty in understanding why there is a high level of concern at the amount of judicial time and public funds spent to keep DOLS alive, when they seem to be 'of little benefit to society'.[83] The DOLS was implemented to protect mentally disabled adults from arbitrary detention to institutional care, unfortunately, this is not the outcome that has materialised.

WORD COUNT - 3,938
(excluding question title and footnotes, including subheadings)

---

[82] Jones, R., *Mental Health Act Manual* (11th ed), (Sweet and Maxwell, 2008).
[83] Lennard, C., 'Deprivation of Liberty Safeguards: complexity, confusion and case law - a commentary' (2014) *5 Social Care and Neurodisability 4*, 245-255, 250.

BIBLIOGRAPHY

Journal Articles

Allen, N., 'Restricting Movement or Depriving Liberty?' (2009) *Journal of Mental Health Law*.

Allen, N., 'The Bournewood Gap (As Amended?)' (2010) *Med Law Rev 18*, 78-85.

Aziz, V.M., Laidlow, R., and Neale, J., 'Implication of changes in Mental Health Laws in 2009-2010, a local Welsh experience' (2013) *Journal of Forensic and Legal Medicine 20, 312-315.*

Banner, N., 'The Bournewood Gap and the Deprivation of Liberty Safeguards in the Mental Capacity Act 2005' (2011) *18 Philosophy, Psychiatry, & Psychology 2, 123-126.*

Blamires, K., Forrester-Jones, R., and Murphy, G., 'An Investigation into the use of the Deprivation of Liberty Safeguards with People with Intellectual Disabilities' (2017) *Journal of Applied Research in Intellectual Disabilities 30, 714-726.*

Cairns, R., *et al*, 'Mired in confusion: making sense of the Deprivation of Liberty Safeguards' (2011) *51 Med Sci Law 4, 228–236.*

Campbell, A., 'Interpreting the Deprivation of Liberty Safeguards legislation' (2014) *16 NRC 1.*

Clements, 'Disability, Dignity and the cri de coeur' (2011) *EHRLR 675.*

Dwyer, S., 'The Deprivation of Liberty Safeguards and People with Dementia: Implications for Social Workers' (2010) British Journal of Social Work 40, 1503-1516.

Elliot, T., 'Commentary: Deprivation of Liberty and the Mental Capacity Act 2005' (2011) *19 Medical Law Rev 1, 132-139.*

Fanning, J., 'Continuities of risk in the era of the Mental Capacity Act' (2016) *24 Medical Law Rev 3, 415-433.*

Fennell, P., 'Doctor Knows Best? Therapeutic detention under Common Law, the Mental Health Act, and the European Convention' (1998) *Med Law Rev 6*, 322-353.

Fovargue, S., Miola, J., 'Assessing and detaining those who are mentally disordered under the Mental Health Act 1983 and Mental Capacity Act 2005: Part 1' (2011) *Clinical Ethics 6, 11-14.*

Frankova, H., 'Deprivation of Liberty Safeguards: a gilded cage is still a cage' (2015) *17 NRC 3.*

Hargraves, R., 'The Deprivation of Liberty Safeguards – essential protection or bureaucratic monster?' (Winter 2009) *Journal of Mental Health Law*.

Keene, A.R., 'Mental Capacity Report: Special Report: the Law Commission's Mental Capacity and Deprivation of Liberty Report (Law Com No. 372)' (2017) *39 Essex Chambers*.

Keene, A.R:, 'Tying ourselves into (Gordian) knots? – deprivation of liberty and the MCA 2005' (2013) *3 Elder Law Journal 1, 69.*

Keywood, K., 'Detaining Mentally Disordered Patients Lacking Capacity: The arbitrariness of informal detention and the common law doctrine of necessity' (2005) *Med Law Rev.*

Lennard, C., 'Deprivation of Liberty Safeguards (DoLS) - where do we go from here?' (2015) *17 Journal of Adult Protection 1*, 41-50.

Lennard, C., 'Deprivation of Liberty Safeguards: complexity, confusion and case law - a commentary' (2014) *5 Social Care and Neurodisability 4*, 245-255.

Lepping, P., Sambhi, R.S., Williams-Jones, K., 'Deprivation of liberty safeguards: how prepared are we?' (2010) *J Med Ethics 36, 170-173*

McKillop, M., *et al*, 'The concept of objection under the DOLS regime' (2011) *Journal of Mental Health Law 61.*

Pearce, N., and Jackson., S., 'Deprivation of Liberty Safeguards Part 2: the Authorisation Regime: statutory provisions of authorisations and Code of Practice' (April, 2012) *Fam Law 432.*

Pearce, N., and Jackson., S., 'Deprivation of Liberty Safeguards Part 3: how the authorisation regime safeguards are working' (May, 2012) *Fam Law 567.*

Pearce, N., and Jackson., S., 'Deprivation of Liberty Safeguards Part 5: general jurisdiction and role of the Court of Protection' (July, 2012) *Fam Law 851.*

Pearce, N., and Jackson., S., 'Deprivation of Liberty Safeguards Part 6: definition of deprivation of liberty' (August, 2012) Fam Law 999.

Phull, J.S., 'The Deprivation of Liberty Safeguards: observations and limitations' (2011) *Med Sci Law 51, 187-192.*

Richardson, 'Mental capacity at the margin: the interface between two Acts' (2010) *18 Medical Law Review 1, 56.*

Robinson, R., Scott-Moncrieff, L., 'Making Sense of Bournewood' (2005) *J. Mental Health L. 17.*

Selmes, T., Robinson, J., Mills, E., Branton, T. and Barlow, J., "Prevalence of deprivation of liberty: a survey of in-patient services" (2010) *34 The Psychiatrist 6*, 221-5.

Shah, A., 'Review Article: Implications of a new case law on the Deprivation of Liberty Safeguards' (2010) Med Sci Law 50.

Shah, A., Heginbotham, C., and Kinton, M., 'The Legal Authority to 'More Than Merely Restrain' Incapacitated Patients: The Interface Between the Mental Capacity Act and the Revised Mental Health Act in England And Wales' (2009) *14 Mental Health Review Journal 1.*

Stewart, R., 'Letter' (2006) *British Medical Journal 332.*

Tingle, J., 'Deprivation of liberty safeguards: a human rights issue' (2012) 21 *British Journal of Nursing 9.*

Tingle, J., The use of the Mental Capacity Act Deprivation of Liberty Safeguards' (2013) *22 British Journal of Nursing 12.*

Troke, B., 'The death of deprivation of liberty safeguards?' (2012) *3 Social Care and Neurodisability 2.*

Yoemans, P., 'Deprivation of Liberty Safeguards: Living DOLS' (2012) *6 British Journal of Healthcare Assistants 9.*

Books
Bartlett, P., and Sandland, R., *Mental Health Law: Policy and Practice* (4th ed) (OUP, 2013).

Jackson, E., *Medical Law: Texts, Cases and Materials* (5th ed) (OUP, 2019).

Jones, R., *Mental Health Act Manual* (11th ed), (Sweet and Maxwell, 2008).

Titterton, M., *Risk and Risk Taking in Health and Social Welfare*, (London, Jessica Kingsley, 2005).

Law Commission Reports
Law Commission Report, Mental Incapacity (Law Com No. 231) [1995]

Government Reports and Codes of Practice
House of Lords Paper 139, *Select Committee on the Mental Capacity Act 2005*, 'Mental Capacity Act 2005: post-legislative scrutiny' Report of Session 2013–14.

Mental Capacity Act 2005: Code of Practice (2007) (TSO, London).

European Conventions
European Convention of Human Rights

UK Legislation
Mental Capacity Act 2005
Mental Health Act 1983
Mental Health Act 2007

Case Law
Cheshire West and Chester Council v P [2011] EWCA Civ 1257
Cheshire West and Chester Council v P [2014] UKSC 19, [2014] MHLO 16
F v West Berkshire Health Authority and another [1989] 2 All ER 545.
R. v Bournewood Community and Mental Health NHS Trust Ex p. L [1998] UKHL 24

EU Case Law
Guzzardi v Italy (Application no. 7367/76) [1981] 3 E.H.R.R. 333.
HL v The United Kingdom [2004] (2005) 40 EHRR 32.
Stanev v Bulgaria (Application No. 36760/06) [2012] ECHR 46
Winterwerp v the Netherlands (Application No. 6301/73) [1979] 2 EHRR 387.

Online Resources
Department of Health and Social Care, Mental Capacity (Amendment) Bill, Impact Assessment (29/06/2018) <https://publications.parliament.uk/pa/bills/lbill/2017-2019/0117/mental-capacity-IA.pdf> (Accessed June 2020).

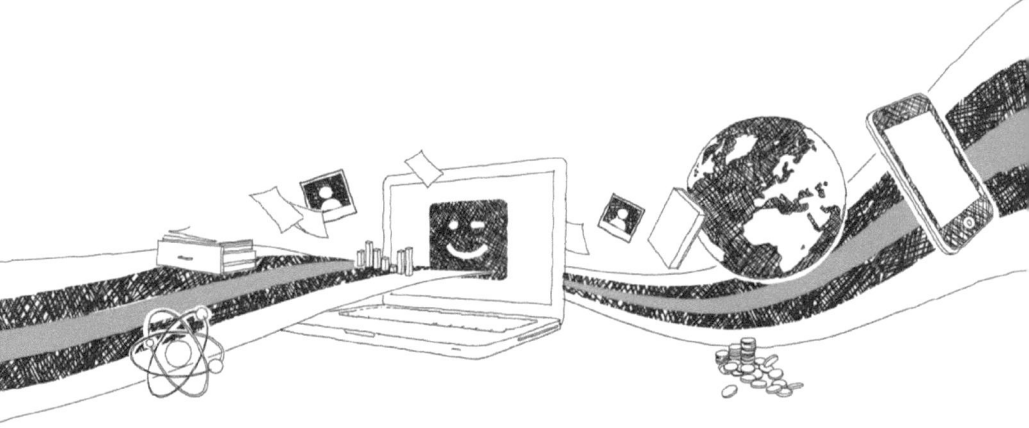
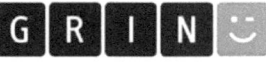